ICS 11.202

SCM

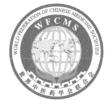

世界中医药学会联合会
World Federation of Chinese Medicine Societies

SCM 0050-2019

国际中医远程教育服务规范

Specifications for International Chinese Medicine
Distance Learning Service

U0319404

世界中联国际组织标准   2019-12-26发布实施
International Standard of WFCMS   Issued & implemented on December 26th, 2019

中医古籍出版社
Publishing House of Ancient Chinese Medical Books

图书在版编目（CIP）数据

国际中医远程教育服务规范：汉英对照 / 世界中医
药学会联合会著 . —北京：中医古籍出版社，2020.7

ISBN 978-7-5152-2147-2

Ⅰ . ①国… Ⅱ . ①世… Ⅲ . ①中医教育—远程教育—
社会服务—规范—汉、英 Ⅳ . ① R2-4

中国版本图书馆 CIP 数据核字（2020）第 126306 号

国际中医远程教育服务规范

世界中医药学会联合会　著

责任编辑　王晓曼

特约编辑　张　楚

出版发行　中医古籍出版社有限公司

社　　址　北京东直门内南小街 16 号（100700）

电　　话　010-64089446（总编室）010-64002949（发行部）

网　　址　www.zhongyiguji.com.cn

印　　刷　北京建宏印刷有限公司

开　　本　880mm×1230mm　1/16

印　　张　1.75

字　　数　54 千字

版　　次　2020 年 7 月第 1 版　2020 年 7 月第 1 次印刷

书　　号　ISBN 978-7-5152-2147-2

定　　价　36.00 元

目　　次

前　　言

本标准主要起草单位：

中　　国：江苏省中医院（南京中医药大学附属医院）

本标准参与起草单位：

美　　国：克利夫兰州立大学、洛杉矶中医药大学

加 拿 大：加拿大多伦多华助中心

英　　国：英国兰维多利亚学院

泰　　国：泰国曼谷市华侨报德善堂附属华侨中医院

巴　　西：巴西华助中心

奥 地 利：奥地利卡尔兰斯坦科研所

本标准主要起草人：

中　　国：吴文忠、束雅春、龚秀琴、张犁、李晓云、陈理

本标准参与起草人：

美　　国：王蜀、Yan Xu

加 拿 大：John Li、金涛、刘莉莉、郑永麟

英　　国：汤淑兰

泰　　国：徐慧兰

巴　　西：刘皓、张伟

奥 地 利：李宏颖

本标准的起草程序遵守了世界中医药学会联合会发布的《世界中医药学会联合会国际组织标准管理办法》。

本标准由世界中医药学会联合会发布，版权归世界中医药学会联合会所有。

国际中医远程教育服务规范

1 范围

本文件规定了国际中医远程教育服务的服务提供者、服务人员、服务资源、工作流程、服务评价与改进措施等方面的要求。

本文件适用于国际中医远程教育服务的管理、实施与评价。

2 规范性引用文件

下列文件对于本文件的应用是必不可少的。凡是注日期的引用文件，仅注日期的版本适用于本文件。凡是不注日期的引用文件，其最新版本（包括所有的修改单）适用于本文件。

GB/T 21644−2008 网络远程教育平台总体要求

GB/T 26997−2011 非正规教育与培训的学习服务术语

GB/T 35273−2017 信息安全技术个人信息安全规范

SCM 0003−2009 世界中医本科（CMD 前）教育标准

SCM 0010−2012 世界中医学专业核心课程

3 术语和定义

下列术语和定义适用于本文件。

3.1
国际中医远程教育服务

利用卫星、计算机、多媒体、网络技术、移动技术等，开展远距离、跨境的中医远程教育，学习中医药理论、基本技能、中医临床运用等为核心的活动的集合。

3.2
服务提供者

提供中医远程教育服务的组织、机构。

3.3
受众

包括学员和购买机构两个部分。

3.4
学员

接受国际中医远程教育服务的个人，包括世界范围的中医药从业者、中医药培训者、想获取中医药知识者以及希望通过远程教育获得中医药专业学历者。

注： 改写 GB/T 26997–2011.定义 2.4。

3.5
购买机构

购买国际中医远程教育服务的单位或组织。

3.6
教学人员

在国际中医远程教育服务中，指导学员开展学习活动的专业授课人员。

注： 改写 GB/T 26997–2011.定义 4.1。

3.7
教辅人员

在国际中医远程教育服务中，为教学人员和学员提供支持服务的相关人员。

示例：

教学设计人员、信息技术支持人员、管理人员、语言支持人员。

注： 改写 GB/T 26997–2011.定义 4.2。

4 国际中医远程教育工作流程

4.1 协议订立

4.1.1 服务提供者应与受众订立服务协议。

4.1.2 服务协议应包括服务内容、服务时间与地点、全部费用及明细、服务变更手续、投诉与纠纷解决方法、隐私保护、风险提示，以及双方权利义务、法律责任等内容，同时应对影响服务质量的其他关键要素进行约定。

4.1.3 服务协议应体现公平、公正的原则，在双方平等、自愿的前提下订立。

4.1.4 服务提供者应履行告知义务，提醒受众注意协议中与其利益密切相关的内容，告知形式包括口头告知、电子信息告知、书面告知、公示告知等。

4.2 方案确定

4.2.1 服务提供者应对受众的需求进行了解，确定服务目标。

示例：

学员的学习目标、希望获得的学习效果、原本具备的中医水平、语言情况及希望远程教育服务所采用的方式、服务时间等。

4.2.2 服务提供者应对学员的专业基础、教育经历以及现有水平等进行了解。

4.2.3 依据服务目标为受众选择或设计中医远程教育的服务内容、服务方式、服务时间等，形成服务方案。

4.2.4 服务方案的内容和实施条件应得到受众认可。

4.3 开展中医远程教育活动

4.3.1 服务提供者的资质应符合所在国相关要求。

4.3.2 服务提供者应根据服务方案提供与国际中医远程教育服务匹配的服务资源，建立服务管理制度并有效实施，按照服务协议开展国际中医远程教育服务活动。

5 国际中医远程教育服务管理细则

5.1 机构管理

开展国际中医远程教育服务的机构应当按照以下要求开展工作：

5.1.1 结合本国国情，制定并落实教育管理规章制度。

5.1.2 设置专门的教学质量管理部门或配备专职管理人员，负责国际中医远程教育服务质量管理与控制工作，履行以下职责：

——对各项规章制度、教学规范等的落实情况进行检查；

——对教学质量、信息系统和设备管理等方面进行检查；

——对重点环节和影响教学质量因素进行监测、分析和反馈，提出预防与控制措施。

5.1.3 服务信息提供

5.1.3.1 服务提供者应为受众提供相关服务信息，主要包括：

——教学、教辅人员基本情况；

——线上中医药学习的安排；

——所采用的学习资源；

——全部费用明细、支付方式；

——服务变更手续；

——参与学习活动应具备的条件；

——服务承诺和风险提示。

5.1.3.2 提供相关事宜的信息咨询服务，咨询渠道方便、快捷、畅通。

5.1.3.3 服务信息应真实、准确、完整，具有时效性，与实际服务一致。

5.2 人员管理

5.2.1 教学人员

5.2.1.1 专业知识要求

教学人员应具备中医药专业知识、远程教育信息系统使用知识，在本国法律框架下具备相应教育资质及授课能力。

5.2.1.2 教学活动设计能力

——教学人员根据受众需求进行分析，有针对性地编写教学大纲，确定教学方案；
——教学方案应说明学习的目的和要求，明确学习知识和技能方面的预期效果；
——以学员为中心设计服务方式与形式；
——设计符合中医药教学特点的学习活动；
——选择适当的评价方法和评价标准。

5.2.1.3 教学活动组织能力

——选择优质学习资源，并通过合适的渠道、方式，推送至受众；
——设置适当的学习任务，明确重点掌握的内容，关注学习过程并提供反馈；
——确定学习难点，理解学员的问题与需求，提供有效辅导或线上咨询解答；
——鼓励学员参与学习和相关讨论。
示例：
通过视频会议、直播平台等形式进行讨论、示范操作、中医试诊、测试考核，组织开展中医药知识教学活动。

5.2.1.4 教学评估能力

——教学人员应能够收集有关信息，准确分析、评估学习活动情况，及时发现问题与不足并加以改进；
——教学人员利用信息技术手段，应具有形成性评估和终结性评估的能力。

5.2.1.5 信息技术应用能力

——掌握远程教育信息系统基本使用方法，以合适、多样的方式呈现教学内容；
——能运用信息技术促进学员有效学习。

5.2.2 教辅人员

5.2.2.1 教辅人员应具备有效支持国际中医远程教育活动顺利开展的职业能力。
5.2.2.2 根据工作内容不同，教辅人员应具备以下能力中的一项或多项：
——协助教学人员进行课件制作、学习环境设计（线上教学设备、教具等）、组织小组讨论等能力；
——掌握并运用远程教育信息系统的基本方法，为学员提供相应帮助；
——具有与中医药学习活动有关的咨询能力、反馈能力；
——沟通交流能力。

5.2.2.3 语言服务支持人员

如需外语教学，服务方配备1名熟练运用该国语言的教学人员或翻译人员。

5.3 教学资源管理

5.3.1 学习平台

学习平台包括 Web 学习平台、App 学习平台、虚拟仿真实验室、直播教学平台等。

5.3.1.1 学习平台设备应满足

——符合 GB/T 21644 要求；
——功能完善，满足教学、学习、教辅服务需求；
——信息安全且传输有效；
——具有可靠性、稳定性。

5.3.1.2 学习平台功能要求

根据各国远程教学信息系统实施方式的异同，其学习平台应根据需求选择具备以下多项功能：

——在线报名、缴费、注册；
——受众信息登记、管理；
——在线选课、视频点播、即时音频或视频通话；
——在线课程学习、在线授课、实时和非实时在线答疑；
——讨论、任务协作；
——学习资源共享、下载、查看、播放；
——课程调整等教务管理；
——学习情况统计等教学管理；
——投诉、辅导、技术保障等支持服务。

5.3.1.3 学习平台应提供便捷的远程教育服务。

5.3.1.4 学员可通过多种设备（移动端、PC 端）访问和使用学习资源。

5.3.2 课程设置

5.3.2.1 服务提供者应围绕学员的需求设置课程。中医学专业核心课程可参照 SCM 0010-2012 标准。

5.3.2.2 服务提供者可根据不同国家、地区学员需求，提供针对性及个性化的课程。

5.3.2.3 在设置课程时，服务提供者应将在线教学工具及使用方式纳入其中，帮助学员在线学习。

5.3.2.4 服务提供者应注重课程设置的合理性、系统性，方便学员选择与远程学习。

5.3.3 教学资料

教学资料包括文本型、图片型、音 / 视频型学习资源及多媒体素材等。

5.3.3.1 教学资料中的文字、图片、音 / 视频等信息应与教学内容协调、一致。

5.3.3.2 教学资料应具有科学性、专业性、适用性。

——符合中医学专业学习特点和认知规律；
——综合运用中医临床案例教学。

示例：

充分运用教学资源，可开展中医理论学习，中医理、法、方、药的运用与临床实施，针灸、推拿等中医适宜技术示范操作等学习。

5.3.3.3 根据学习目标，匹配与教学内容相一致的测试与考核资料，开展教学评估。

5.3.3.4 教学资料不应在性别、年龄、种族、宗教等方面存在偏见。

5.3.3.5 使用的教学软件应适用于学习平台并及时更新，各更新版本应方便学员获取。

5.4 教学质量管理

5.4.1 教学管理人员督促落实各项规章制度和日常远程教学管理工作，并对本机构中医远程教育服务行为进行检查。

5.4.2 教学人员应严格按照教学方案进行教学活动，不可随意删减教学内容、缩短教学时间。

5.4.3 教辅人员应始终围绕教学目标，协助教学人员做好教学服务工作，根据需求开展指导、答疑、讨论、咨询、作业批改与反馈等服务。

5.4.4 信息技术人员做好中医远程医疗设备、信息系统的日常维护，保证其正常运转。

6 安全要求

6.1 应用安全

学习平台应通过完备设置认证机制、分级权限管理、操作日志等方式，保证应用安全。

6.2 网络安全

服务提供者应采取措施，维护学习平台网络环境的安全性，有预防信息数据泄密、系统破坏等的应急预案。

6.3 数据安全

6.3.1 服务提供者应建立受众信息管理制度，按照GB/T35273要求管理受众信息。

6.3.2 在受众知情同意的前提下，收集、统计或使用相关信息。

6.3.3 服务提供者应采取措施，维护学习平台上受众信息，包括个人隐私等数据安全，防止其信息泄露、丢失。禁止任何人以出售等形式非法向他人提供受众信息。

示例：

数据库安全策略、敏感数据存储和传输加密、数据备份和恢复机制。

6.3.4 服务提供者应根据数据备份策略定期对教学服务数据进行备份、转储，资料完整、真实、准确。

7 费用支付

7.1 服务提供者应确保实际服务交付的内容与服务协议约定的一致。

7.2 服务提供者应向受众说明支付的有关信息并达成一致，主要包括：

——全部费用及明细；

——支付方式；

——支付出现问题时的解决措施。

7.3 服务提供者应为受众提供多种支付方式，当选用某种支付方式将产生额外费用时，应在支付前向受众说明。

7.4 在支付完成后，向受众提供支付凭证。

8 教学评估

8.1 服务提供者应在教学过程中和完成后，分别对学员的学习效果进行形成性评估和终结性评估，判断教学目标的完成情况并及时调整。

8.2 评估内容主要包括：

——学员在各方面学习发展水平与所约定服务目标的比对情况；

——学员在学习活动中的表现；

——学员对于学习平台、学习资源等的适应性。

8.3 评估方法主要包括观察、交流、测试、调查等。

8.4 评估结果能真实反映学员学习效果。

9 评价与改进

9.1 国际中医远程教育机构应建立服务评价管理机制，可接受相关人员和部门的评价。

9.2 服务评价应：

——具备科学的评价方案，评价行为依据评价方案开展；

——对所采集的真实数据进行分析，得出评价结果，评价结果能客观、准确地反映评价活动情况，具有高信度。

9.3 评价者应根据不同评价目标，可参见附录A，从中选取合适的评价指标并进行细化、组合、赋权，建立评价指标体系，实施具体评价活动。

9.4 服务提供者应根据服务评价结果，提出预防与控制措施，制定整改方案，持续改进，不断提高服务水平。

10 教育证书

10.1 对于攻读中医药相关学历的学员，可参考各国相应的教育标准，采取线上与线下学习相结合的方式，结合学历教育考核评价体系，完成全部核心课程及临床实践者可颁发相应学历教育证书。

示例：

攻读本科的学生，可参考SCM 0003-2009世界中医本科（CMD前）教育标准。

10.2 对于参加中医药非学历教育的学员，接受中医远程教育服务，参加线上短期培训的学员，根据学习完成情况，提供学习证明。

附录 A

（规范性附录）

国际中医远程教育服务评价指标

国际中医远程教育服务评价指标如表 A.1 所示。

表 A.1 国际中医远程教育服务评价指标

序号	一级指标	二级指标
1	中医远程教育服务流程	服务提供者与受众订立服务协议
2		服务协议内容全面
3		服务提供者在与受众订立服务协议之前履行告知义务
4		服务提供者了解受众需求与特征，确定服务方案
5		服务方案内容符合要求并得到受众认可
6		提供的服务资源与国际中医远程服务相一致
7	教育服务机构管理	制定并落实相关教育管理规章制度
8		配备专职管理人员、教学人员、教辅人员
9		提供的服务信息真实、准确、完整
10		服务信息符合国际中医远程教育要求
11	教学人员管理	教学人员资质符合要求
12		教学人员具有教学活动设计、组织、信息技术应用等能力
13		教学人员能定期进行教学效果评估
14	教辅人员管理	教辅人员按要求开展一切教辅活动，能满足教学人员及学员要求
15		根据工作内容不同，完成各自的教辅任务：协助组织各种教学活动、教具准备、环境准备、信息技术支持等
16		能提供教学咨询、教学反馈
17		沟通能力强
18	学习平台管理	学习平台满足学习、教学、教辅需求，符合 GB/T 21644 等标准要求
19		学习平台信息系统安全、稳定
20		学习平台与学习活动内容与形式相适应
21		学习平台使用方便

序号	一级指标	二级指标
22	课程设置要求	课程设置围绕受众需求
23		课程设置满足不同国家、地区的个性化要求
24		课程设置合理、系统
25	教学资料要求	教学资料符合中医药专业的学习特点和认知规律，通俗易懂，科普性强
26		教学资料中的文字、图片、音／视频等符合教学内容，教学软件适用于学习平台
27		教学资料无性别、年龄、种族、宗教等偏见
28		有与教学内容相匹配的测试、考核资料
29	教学过程质量管理	质量管理人员督促落实各项制度
30		质量管理人员定期对日常教学、教辅服务进行检查
31		教学内容、课时安排符合教学方案
32		教辅支持满足教学要求
33	安全要求	教育机构有受众信息管理制度并落实
34		应在受众知情、许可的前提下，收集、使用受众信息，信息完整
35		学习平台设置认证机制、分级管理权限，保证应用安全
36		学习平台网络环境安全
37		有保护受众信息、隐私安全应对措施
38		无出售等形式非法向他人提供受众信息
39		教学数据适时备份、转储，资料完整、准确、真实
40	服务费用支付	服务提供者向受众说明全部费用及明细、支付方式、支付出现问题时的解决措施
41		服务提供者为受众提供多种支付方式
42		当产生额外费用时，服务提供者在支付前向受众说明
43		支付完成后，向支付方提供支付凭证
44	学习效果评估	服务提供者在学习活动过程中，对学员的学习进行形成性评估
45		服务提供者能根据服务目标的完成情况，开展教学评估
46		评估方法多样
47	服务评价与改进	有针对国际中医远程教育服务的评价管理机制
48		建立合理的评价体系，实施具体评价活动
49		评价方案科学，可操作
50		采集数据真实，评价结果客观、准确，具有高信度
51		服务提供机构能根据评价结果，就存在问题制定整改措施，持续改进，有记录
52	教育证书	根据不同学员的学习目标与考核标准，给符合要求的学员颁发教育证书或学习证明

Foreword

Main drafting organization: Jiangsu Provincial Hospital of Chinese Traditional Medicine (Affiliated Hospital of Nanjing University of Chinese Traditional Medicine)

Drafting organizations participated:
USA: Cleveland State University, Los Angeles Chinese Medicine University
Canada: Toronto Overseas Chinese Service Center
UK: Shulan College of Chinese UK
Thailand: Hua Chiew Chinese Medicine Hospital, Poh Teck Tung Foundation, Bangkok
Brazil: Overseas Chinese Service Center
Austria: Association for the Promotion of Medical-Scientific Research

Main Drafters:
China: Wu Wenzhong, Shu Yachun, Gong Xiuqin, Zhang Li, Li Xiaoyun, Chen Li

Drafters and reviewers:
USA: Wang Shu, Yan Xu
Canada: John Li, Jin Tao, Liu Lili, Zheng Yonglin
UK: Tang Shulan
Thailand: Xu Huilan
Brazil: Liu Hao, Zhang Wei
Austria: Li Hongying

The drafting procedures of this Standard conform to the SCM 0001-2009 *Specifications on Standard Formulation and Publishing* issued by World Federation of Chinese Medicine Societies.

This standard is issued by WFCMS, and all copyrights are reserved to WFCMS.

Specifications for International Chinese Medicine Distance Learning Service

1 Scope

This standard specifies the requirements for service providers, service personnel, service resources, procedures, service evaluation and measures for improvement, etc. in international Chinese medicine distance learning service.

This standard shall be applicable to the management, implementation and evaluation of international Chinese medicine distance learning service.

2 Normative References

The following documents are necessary for the application of this document. For dated references, only their dated versions are applicable to this document. For undated references, their latest versions (including all the amendments) are applicable to this document.

GB/T 21644-2008 General Description of Networks Distance Learning

GB/T 26997-2011 Learning Services for Non-formal Education and Training — Terminology

GB/T 35273-2017 Information Security Technology — Personal Information Security Specification

SCM 0003-2009 World Standard of Chinese Medicine Undergraduate (pre-CMD) Education

SCM 0010-2012 World Core Courses of Chinese Medicine Specialty

3 Terms and Definitions

For the purposes of this document, the following terms and definitions apply.

3.1 International Chinese Medicine Distance Learning Service

A series of activities focused on long-distance and cross-border learning of Chinese medicine-related theories, basic skills and clinical application and carried out with satellites, computers, multimedia, network technology, mobile technology, etc.

3.2 Providers of Chinese Medicine Distance Learning Service

Organizations and institutions that provide Chinese medicine distance learning service (hereinafter referred to as "service providers").

3.3 Service Recipients

Learners and purchasing organizations.

3.4 Learners

Individuals that accept international Chinese medicine distance learning service, including worldwide practitioners of Chinese medicine, trainees of Chinese medicine, people who want to acquire Chinese medicine knowledge and professional qualifications in Chinese medicine through distance learning.

Note: A revised version of Definition 2.4 of GB/T 26997-2011.

3.5 Purchasing Organizations

Units or organizations that purchase international Chinese medicine distance learning service.

3.6 Faculty Members

Professional instructors that instruct the learners' learning activities in international Chinese medicine distance learning service.

Note: A revised version of Definition 4.1 of GB/T 26997-2011.

3.7 Supporting Staff

Relevant personnel that provide supporting services for faculty members and learners in international Chinese medicine distance learning service.

Examples:

instructional designers, technical support staff, administrators, personnel providing translation or interpreting services.

Note: A revised version of Definition 4.2 of GB/T 26997-2011.

4 Process of International Chinese Medicine Distance Learning Service

4.1 Signing Service Agreements

4.1.1 Service providers shall sign service agreements with the service recipients.

4.1.2 The service agreements shall include the service content, service time and location, total expenses and details, procedures for service changes, complaint and dispute settlement, privacy protection, risk disclosure, as well as the rights, obligations and legal duties of both parties. Meanwhile, other key elements that affect service quality shall be agreed upon by both parties.

4.1.3 The service agreements shall be signed on the principle of fairness and justice and under the premise of equality and free will of both parties.

4.1.4 The service providers shall perform the duty of disclosure, and inform the recipients of the contents in the agreements that are closely related to their interests. The forms of disclosure include oral notification, notification with electronic information, written notification, public notification, etc.

4.2 Confirming Service Plans

4.2.1 Service providers shall understand the demands of the recipients so as to identify the service objectives.

Examples:

the learners' learning objectives, the outcomes they hope to achieve, their level of understanding of Chinese medicine and languages, and their desired approach, form and service time of the distance learning service, etc.

4.2.2 Service providers shall know about the learners' professional basis, education background, and current level of expertise, etc.

4.2.3 Choose or design service contents, approaches and time of Chinese medicine distance learning for recipients according to the service objectives to form service plans.

4.2.4 The contents and conditions for implementation of the service plans shall be acknowledged by the recipients.

4.3 Carrying Out Chinese Medicine Distance Learning Activities

4.3.1 The qualifications of service providers shall comply with the relevant requirements of the host country.

4.3.2 Service providers shall provide service resources that are suitable for international Chinese medicine distance learning service according to the service plans, establish and effectively implement the service management system, and carry out international Chinese medicine distance learning activities in accordance with the service agreements.

5 Management Rules of Chinese Medicine Distance Learning Service

5.1 Management of Institutions

Institutions providing international Chinese medicine distance learning service shall operate according to the following requirements:

5.1.1 Formulate and implement the education management regulations based on the national conditions of their host countries.

5.1.2 Set up a special department of teaching quality management or appoint specially-assigned personnel to manage and control the quality of international Chinese medicine distance learning service and perform the following duties:

— Examine the implementation of all the rules, regulations, teaching norms, etc.

— Examine the teaching quality, information system, equipment management, etc.

— Inspect, analyze and give feedback on important steps and influencing factors of teaching quality, and put forward precautions and controlling measures.

5.1.3 Provide service information

5.1.3.1 Service providers shall provide the recipients with relevant service information, mainly including:

— Basic information of faculty members and supporting staff;

— Arrangement of online Chinese medicine study;

— Learning resources that are used;

— Details and payment method of total expense;

— Procedures for service changes;

— Prerequisite conditions for participating in learning activities;

— Service commitment and risk disclosure.

5.1.3.2 Provide information consulting service on related issues, and maintain convenient, efficient and open channels for consultation.

5.1.3.3 Service information shall be true, accurate, complete, up-to-date, and consistent with the actual service.

5.2 Personnel Management

5.2.1 Faculty Members

5.2.1.1 Requirements of professional knowledge

Faculty members shall have professional knowledge of Chinese medicine and knowledge on the operation of distance learning information system, possess corresponding educational qualifications within the framework of domestic laws and be capable of giving lessons.

5.2.1.2 Ability to design learning activities

— Faculty members shall analyze the demands of the recipients, design targeted syllabus and determine the teaching scheme;

— The teaching scheme shall clearly state the purpose and requirements of distance learning to specify the desired effects of studying knowledge and skills;

— Design learner-centered approach and form of service;

— Design learning activities that accord with the characteristics of Chinese medicine teaching;

— Choose proper evaluation methods and criteria.

5.2.1.3 Ability to organize learning activities

— Be capable to choose high quality learning resources, and send them to recipients through appropriate channels and in appropriate ways;

— Set proper learning tasks, determine the key contents, pay attention to the process of learning and give feedback;

— Determine the difficulties in the learning activities, understand the problems and demands of the learners, and provide effective coaching or online consulting;

— Encourage learners to participate in learning activities and relevant discussions.

Examples:

Have discussions, demonstrate operations, make diagnosis, have examinations, and organize learning activities of Chinese medicine knowledge through video conferences, live-streaming platforms, etc.

5.2.1.4 Ability to assess teaching performance

— Faculty members shall be capable to collect relevant information, analyze and assess learning activities accurately, detect the problems and deficiencies in time and improve them;

— Faculty members shall be capable to give formative assessment and summative assessment by means of information technology.

5.2.1.5 Ability to apply information technology

— Command the basic use of the distance learning information system to present the teaching contents in proper and diverse ways;

— Promote learners' effective learning with information technology.

5.2.2 Supporting Staff

5.2.2.1 Supporting staff shall have the vocational ability to effectively support the implementation of international Chinese medicine distance learning activities.

5.2.2.2 According to different work contents, supporting staff shall possess one or more of the following abilities:

— Assist faculty members in courseware making, learning environment design (online teaching equipment, teaching aids, etc.) and organizing group discussions;

— Master and use the basic methods of distance learning information system so as to help learners;

— The ability of consultation and giving feedback that are related to Chinese medicine learning activities;

— Communication skills.

5.2.2.3 Supporting staff of language services

If teaching with foreign languages is required, service providers shall assign 1 faculty member or translator who is proficient in the language of the country.

5.3 Management of Teaching Resources

5.3.1 Learning Platforms

Learning platforms include Web learning platform, App learning platform, virtual simulation laboratory, live-streaming teaching platform, etc.

5.3.1.1 The equipment of learning platforms shall

— meet the requirements of GB/T 21644;

— have complete functions to meet the needs of teaching, learning and teaching assistance services;

— ensure information security and effective transmission;

— be reliable and stable.

5.3.1.2 Functional requirements of the learning platforms

According to the similarities and differences in the implementation of distance learning information systems in different countries, the learning platforms shall have some of the following functions as needed:

— Online application, payment and registration;

— Registration and management of recipients' information;

— Online course selection, video on demand, instant audio or video calls;

— Online course learning, online teaching, real-time and non-real-time online question answering;

— Discussion and task collaboration;

— Sharing, downloading, viewing and playing learning resources;

— Administration of teaching affairs such as curriculum adjustment;

— Teaching management such as learning statistics;

— Support services such as complaints handling, counseling, and technical support.

5.3.1.3 Learning platforms shall provide convenient distance learning services.

5.3.1.4 Learners can get access to and use learning resources through a variety of devices (mobile clients, PCs).

5.3.2 Curriculum Design

5.3.2.1 Service providers shall develop the curriculum according to the needs of the learners. The core courses of Chinese medicine specialty can refer to the standard SCM 0010-2012.

5.3.2.2 Service providers can provide targeted and personalized courses according to the needs of learners from different countries and regions.

5.3.2.3 While developing the curriculum, service providers shall incorporate online teaching tools and methods to help learners study online.

5.3.2.4 Service providers shall make the curriculum more rational and systematic, so as to make it easier for learners to make choices and study by distance learning.

5.3.3 Teaching Materials

Teaching materials include text-based, picture-based, audio/video-based learning resources and multimedia materials.

5.3.3.1 The texts, images, audios/videos and other information in teaching materials shall be coordinated and consistent with the teaching contents.

5.3.3.2 Teaching materials shall be scientific, professional and applicable.

— Conform to the learning characteristics and cognitive rules of Chinese medicine specialty;

— Apply Chinese medicine clinical cases in teaching comprehensively;

Examples:

Make full use of the teaching resources to carry out Chinese medicine theoretical learning, application and clinical implementation of Chinese medicine principles, methods, formulas and medicines, and demonstration of appropriate Chinese medicine technologies such as acupuncture and moxibustion and tuina, etc.

5.3.3.3 According to the learning objectives, provide examination and assessment materials that align with the teaching contents to carry out teaching assessment.

5.3.3.4 Teaching materials shall not be biased in terms of gender, age, race, religion, etc.

5.3.3.5 Teaching software that is used shall be applicable to the learning platforms and be updated in time. The updated versions shall be easy for the learners to obtain.

5.4 Quality Management of Teaching Activities

5.4.1 Teaching managers shall supervise the implementation of the rules and regulations and the daily management of distance learning, and examine the behaviors of the institutions in Chinese medicine distance learning service.

5.4.2 Faculty members shall carry out teaching activities in strict conformity with the teaching scheme, and must not delete teaching contents and shorten teaching time at will.

5.4.3 Supporting staff shall always focus on the teaching objectives, assist faculty members in providing quality service, and give instructions, answer questions, have discussions, offer consultations, correct homework and give feedback as needed.

5.4.4 IT personnel shall be in charge of the daily maintenance of Chinese medicine telemedicine equipment and information system to ensure their normal operation.

6 Security Requirements

6.1 Application Security

The learning platforms shall ensure the application security by setting up a complete authentication mechanism, level-to-level access management, operation logs, etc.

6.2 Network Security

Service providers shall take measures to maintain the network security of the learning platforms, and prepare emergency plans to prevent information and data leakage, system damage, etc.

6.3 Data Security

6.3.1 Service providers shall establish an information management system for the recipients and manage the recipients' information in accordance with the requirements of GB/T35273.

6.3.2 Collect, record or use relevant information with the consent of the recipients.

6.3.3 Service providers shall take measures to maintain the data security of the recipients' information, including personal privacy, on the learning platform to prevent information leakage or loss. Offering the information of the recipients to others in illegal ways, such as selling the information, is strictly forbidden.

Examples:

Database security strategies, encryption of sensitive data storage and transmission, data backup and recovery mechanism.

6.3.4   Service providers shall regularly backup and dump the teaching service data according to the data backup strategies, and the data shall be complete, authentic and accurate.

7   Payment of Charges

7.1   Service providers shall ensure that the content delivered by actual service is consistent with that agreed in the service agreements.

7.2   Service providers shall explain to the recipients the relevant information of the payment and reach an agreement with them, which mainly includes:

— Total expense and details;

— Payment method;

— Solutions to payment problems.

7.3   Service providers shall provide the recipients with a variety of payment methods, and shall explain to the recipients before payment is made when additional fees will be incurred by a certain payment method.

7.4   Payment vouchers shall be offered to the recipients after payment is completed.

8   Assessment of Teaching Performance

8.1   During and after the teaching activities, service providers shall make formative and summative assessment of the learners' learning outcomes respectively to assess the achievement of the teaching objectives and make timely adjustments.

8.2   The assessment mainly includes:

— The comparison between the learners' developmental level in various aspects and the agreed service objectives;

— The learners' performance in learning activities;

— The learners' adaptability to the learning platforms, learning resources, etc.

8.3   The assessment methods mainly include observation, communication, examination, investigation, etc.

8.4   The assessment results should truly reflect the learning outcomes of the learners.

9   Evaluation and Improvement

9.1   International Chinese medicine distance learning institutions shall establish a service evaluation management mechanism, which may accept the evaluation of relevant personnel and departments.

9.2   Service evaluation should

— have a scientific evaluation scheme and conduct evaluation actions based on the evaluation scheme;

— analyze the authentic data collected and produce the evaluation results, which can objectively and accurately reflect the evaluation activities and have high reliability.

9.3 Evaluators should select appropriate evaluation indicators from the Annex A according to different evaluation objectives, and break down, combine and assign scores to them to establish evaluation index system and implement specific evaluation activities.

9.4 Service providers shall put forward precautions and regulatory measures and formulate corrective programs according to service evaluation results to continuously improve service quality.

10 Education Certificates

10.1 Learners who study for Chinese medicine-related diplomas can refer to the corresponding educational standards in different countries, and combine online learning with offline learning based on the diploma assessment and evaluation system. Those who complete all the core courses and clinical practices can be granted with the corresponding education certificates.

Example:

Students studying undergraduate courses can refer to SCM 0003-2009 World Standard of Chinese Medicine Undergraduate (pre-CMD) Education.

10.2 Students who participate in non-diploma Chinese medicine education, Chinese medicine distance learning, and online short-term training will be provided with certificates confirming their learning experience according to their performance and achievements.

Annex A

(Normative Appendix)

International Chinese Medicine Distance Learning Service Evaluation Index

The evaluation index of international Chinese Medicine distance learning service is shown in the following table A.1.

Table A.1 International Chinese Medicine Distance Learning Service Evaluation Index

No.	Primary indicator	Secondary indicator
1	Process of Chinese medicine distance learning service	Service providers sign service agreements with the recipients
2		The contents of the service agreements are comprehensive
3		Service providers perform the duty of disclosure before signing service agreements with the recipients
4		Service Providers confirm the service plan based on the understanding of the demands and characteristics of the recipients
5		The contents of the service plan comply with the requirements and are approved by the recipients
6		The service resources provided are consistent with international Chinese medicine distance learning service
7	Management of Learning Institutions	Formulate and implement relevant education management regulations
8		Be staffed with specially-assigned administrators, faculty members, and supporting staff
9		Provide authentic, accurate and complete service information
10		The service information conforms with the requirements of international Chinese medicine distance learning
11	Management of Faculty Members	The qualification of the faculty members complies with the requirements
12		Faculty members possess the ability to design and organize learning activities, apply information technology, etc.
13		Faculty members can assess learning performance regularly

No.	Primary indicator	Secondary indicator
14	Management of Supporting Staff	Supporting staff carry out all the teaching-related activities as required, and meet the demands of faculty members and learners
15		Complete tasks depending on the different contents of their work: assist in organizing various teaching activities, preparing teaching aids and environment, IT support, etc.
16		Provide teaching consultation and feedback
17		Good communication skills
18	Management of Learning Platforms	Learning platforms meet the needs in learning, teaching and supporting, and accord with the standards of GB/T 21644, etc.
19		The information system of the learning platforms is secure and stable
20		Learning platforms are compatible with the contents and forms of the learning activities
21		Learning platforms are easy to use
22	Requirements for Curriculum Design	The curriculum is designed based on the demands of the recipients
23		The curriculum meets the personalized requirements of different countries and regions
24		The curriculum is rational and systematic
25	Requirements for Teaching Resources	Teaching resources conform to the learning characteristics and cognitive rules of Chinese medicine specialty. They are readily understandable and have a strong function of science popularization
26		The texts, pictures, audios/radios in the teaching resources are consistent with the teaching contents, the teaching software is applicable to the teaching platforms
27		Teaching materials are not biased in terms of gender, age, race, religion, etc.
28		There are examination and assessment materials that match the teaching contents
29	Quality Management of Teaching Activities	Teaching quality managers supervise the implementation of the rules and regulations
30		Teaching quality managers examine daily teaching and teaching assistance services regularly
31		Teaching contents and arrangements of class hours are consistent with the teaching plan
32		Teaching assistance services meet the teaching requirements

No.	Primary indicator	Secondary indicator
33	Security Requirements	Education institutions have implemented management system of recipients' information
34		Collect and use recipients' information with their knowledge and consent, and the information is accurate and complete
35		The learning platforms ensure the application security by setting up a complete authentication mechanism and level-to-level access management
36		The network of the learning platforms is secure
37		There are corrective measures for protecting recipients' information and privacy security
38		There is no illegal offering of recipients' information to others, such as selling the information
39		Backup and dump the teaching data appropriately, and the data shall be complete, authentic and accurate
40	Payment of Service Charges	Service providers explain to recipients the total expense and details, payment methods, and solutions to payment problems
41		Service providers provide recipients with a variety of payment methods
42		Explain to the recipients before payment is made when additional fees will be incurred by a certain payment method
43		Payment vouchers are offered to the recipients after payment is completed
44	Learning Performance Assessment	Service providers give formative assessment to the learners' learning outcomes during the learning activities
45		Service providers carry out learning performance assessment according to the completion of the service objectives
46		The assessment methods are varied
47	Service Evaluation and Improvement	There is a specific evaluation management system for international Chinese medicine distance learning service
48		Establish reasonable evaluation system and implement specific evaluation activities
49		The evaluation scheme is scientific and operable
50		The data collected are authentic, and the evaluation results are objective and accurate with high reliability
51		Institutions that provide services can develop corrective measures for existing problems according to the evaluation results, make continuous improvement and keep a record
52	Education Certificates	Award competent learners with education certificates or proofs of study according to the learning objectives of different learners and evaluation standards